# OBESITY AND WEIGHT LOSS

**Rantho Mahlare MD**

# CONTENT

# WEIGHT AND OBESITY

*Overview*

Weight is a perplexing infection including an extreme measure of muscle to fat ratio. Weight isn't only a corrective concern. It is a clinical issue that expands your danger of different ailments and medical issues, for example, coronary illness, diabetes, hypertension and certain malignancies.

There are numerous reasons why a few people experience issues maintaining a strategic distance from weight. Normally, stoutness results from a blend of acquired variables, joined with the earth and individual eating routine and exercise decisions.

Fortunately, even unobtrusive weight reduction can improve or forestall the medical issues related with heftiness. Dietary changes, expanded physical movement and conduct changes can assist you with shedding pounds. Doctor prescribed drugs and weight reduction methods are extra choices for treating stoutness.

## Key realities

- Worldwide Weight has almost significantly increased since 1975.

- In 2016, more than 1.9 billion grown-ups, 18 years and more established, were Obesity. Of these more than 650 million were large.

- 39% of grown-ups matured 18 years and over were Obesity in 2016, and 13% were corpulent.

- Most of the total populace live in nations where Obesity and Weight murders a bigger number of individuals than underweight.

- 38 million kids younger than 5 were Obesity or large in 2019.

- Over 340 million kids and teenagers matured 5-19 were Obesity or stout in 2016.

- Obesity is preventable.

# WHAT ARE WEIGHT AND OBESITY

Obesity and Weight are characterized as anomalous or exorbitant fat gathering that may weaken wellbeing.

Weight record (BMI) is a straightforward file of weight-for-stature that is normally used to arrange Obesity and Weight in grown-ups. It is characterized as an individual's load in kilograms isolated by the square of his stature in meters (kg/m2).

## Grown-ups

For grown-ups, WHO characterizes Obesity and stoutness as follows:

- Obesity is a BMI more noteworthy than or equivalent to 25; and

- obesity is a BMI more noteworthy than or equivalent to 30.

BMI gives the most helpful populace level proportion of Obesity and stoutness as it is the equivalent for both genders and for all periods of grown-ups. Notwithstanding, it ought to be viewed as an unpleasant guide since it may not relate in a similar way of bloatedness in various people.

For kids, age should be viewed as when characterizing Obesity and Weight.

# Kids under 5 years old

For kids under 5 years old:

- Obesity is weight-for-tallness more noteworthy than 2 standard deviations above WHO Child Growth Standards middle; and

- obesity is weight-for-stature more noteworthy than 3 standard deviations over the WHO Child Growth Standards middle.

- Charts and tables: WHO kid development norms for youngsters matured under 5 years

# Kids matured between 5–19 years

Obesity and stoutness are characterized as follows for youngsters matured between 5–19 years:

- Obesity is BMI-for-age more noteworthy than 1 standard deviation over the WHO Growth Reference middle; and

- obesity is more prominent than 2 standard deviations over the WHO Growth Reference middle.

- Charts and tables: WHO development reference for kids matured between 5–19 years

## Realities about Obesity and Weight

Some ongoing WHO worldwide evaluations follow.

- In 2016, more than 1.9 billion grown-ups matured 18 years and more seasoned were Obesity. Of these more than 650 million grown-ups were corpulent.

- In 2016, 39% of grown-ups matured 18 years and over (39% of men and 40% of ladies) were Obesity.

- Overall, about 13% of the world's grown-up populace (11% of men and 15% of ladies) were stout in 2016.

- The overall predominance of weight almost significantly increased somewhere in the range of 1975 and 2016.

In 2019, an expected 38.2 million kids younger than 5 years were Obesity or large. When considered a high-salary nation issue, Obesity and weight are presently on the ascent in low- and center pay nations, especially in metropolitan settings. In Africa, the quantity of Obesity kids under 5 has expanded by almost 24% percent since 2000. Practically 50% of the kids under 5 who were Obesity or large in 2019 lived in Asia.

More than 340 million kids and young people matured 5-19 were Obesity or hefty in 2016.

The commonness of Obesity and heftiness among kids and young people matured 5-19 has risen significantly from only 4% in 1975 to simply over 18% in 2016. The ascent has happened comparably among the two young men and young ladies: in 2016 18% of young ladies and 19% of young men were Obesity.

While just shy of 1% of youngsters and teenagers matured 5-19 were corpulent in 1975, more 124 million kids and youths (6% of young ladies and 8% of young men) were hefty in 2016.

Obesity and weight are connected to a bigger number of passing's worldwide than underweight. Universally there are a larger number of individuals who are hefty than underweight – this happens in each district aside from parts of sub-Saharan Africa and Asia.

## What causes heftiness and Obesity?

The central reason for Weight and Obesity is a vitality awkwardness between calories devoured and calories consumed. Internationally, there has been:

- an expanded admission of vitality thick nourishments that are high in fat and sugars; and

- an increment in physical dormancy because of the undeniably stationary nature of numerous types of work, changing methods of transportation, and expanding urbanization.

Changes in dietary and physical movement designs are frequently the consequence of ecological and cultural changes related with improvement and absence of strong approaches in segments, for example, wellbeing, horticulture, transport, metropolitan arranging, condition, food handling, appropriation, advertising, and instruction.

## What are normal wellbeing outcomes of Obesity and stoutness?

Raised BMI is a significant danger factor for noncommunicable sicknesses, for example,

- cardiovascular sicknesses (for the most part coronary illness and stroke), which were the main source of death in 2012;

- diabetes;

- musculoskeletal messes (particularly osteoarthritis – an exceptionally debilitating degenerative sickness of the joints);

- some tumors (counting endometrial, bosom, ovarian, prostate, liver, gallbladder, kidney, and colon).

The danger for these noncommunicable ailments increments, with increments in BMI.

Youth heftiness is related with a higher possibility of Weight, unexpected passing and inability in adulthood. Yet, notwithstanding expanded future dangers, large kids experience breathing troubles, expanded danger of breaks, hypertension, early markers of cardiovascular illness, insulin opposition and mental impacts.

## Confronting a twofold weight of unhealthiness

Some low-and center pay nations are currently confronting a "twofold weight" of lack of healthy sustenance.

- While these nations keep on managing the issues of irresistible illnesses and undernutrition, they are additionally encountering a fast upsurge in noncommunicable malady hazard factors, for example, weight and Obesity, especially in metropolitan settings.

- It isn't phenomenal to discover undernutrition and stoutness coinciding inside a similar nation, a similar network and a similar family unit.

Youngsters in low-and center salary nations are more powerless against insufficient pre-natal, baby, and small kid nourishment. Simultaneously, these kids are presented to high-fat, high-sugar, high-salt, vitality thick, and micronutrient-helpless nourishments, which will in general be lower in cost yet additionally lower in supplement quality. These dietary examples, related to bring down degrees of physical action, bring about sharp increments in youth heftiness while undernutrition issues stay unsolved.

## In what capacity can Obesity and stoutness be diminished?

Obesity and Weight, just as their related noncommunicable sicknesses, are generally preventable. Strong conditions and networks are essential in molding individuals' decisions, by settling on the decision of more beneficial nourishments and ordinary physical movement the simplest decision (the decision that is the most open, accessible and reasonable), and in this manner forestalling Obesity and Weight.

At the individual level, individuals can:

- limit vitality admission from all out fats and sugars;
- increase utilization of leafy foods, just as vegetables, entire grains and nuts; and
- engage in customary physical movement (an hour daily for kids and 150 minutes spread during that time for grown-ups).

Singular duty can just have its full impact where individuals approach a solid way of life. Accordingly, at the cultural level it is imperative to help people in following the proposals above, through supported execution of proof based and populace-based arrangements that make normal physical action and more beneficial dietary decisions accessible, moderate and effectively available to everybody, especially to the least fortunate people. A case of such an approach is an assessment on sugar improved refreshments.

The food business can assume a critical part in advancing solid eating regimens by:

- reducing the fat, sugar and salt substance of handled nourishments;

- ensuring that sound and nutritious decisions are accessible and reasonable to all buyers;
- restricting advertising of nourishments high in sugars, salt and fats, particularly those nourishments focused on youngsters and adolescents; and
- ensuring the accessibility of sound food decisions and supporting ordinary physical movement practice in the work environment.

## WHO reaction

Embraced by the World Health Assembly in 2004 and perceived again in a 2011 political announcement on noncommunicable ailment (NCDs), the "WHO Global Strategy on Diet, Physical Activity and Health" depicts the activities expected to help solid eating regimens and standard physical movement. The Strategy calls upon all partners to make a move at worldwide, territorial and neighborhood levels to improve counts calories and physical action designs at the populace level.


The 2030 Agenda for Sustainable Development perceives NCDs as a significant test for practical turn of events. As a major aspect of the Agenda, Heads of State and Government resolved to create aggressive public reactions, by 2030, to diminish by 33% untimely mortality from NCDs through counteraction and treatment (SDG target 3.4).

The "Worldwide activity plan on physical action 2018–2030: more dynamic individuals for a more advantageous world" gives powerful and practical strategy activities to increment physical action internationally. WHO distributed ACTIVE a specialized bundle to help nations in arranging and conveyance of their reactions. New WHO rules on physical action, inactive conduct and rest in youngsters under five years old were dispatched in 2019.

The World Health Assembly invited the report of the Commission on Ending Childhood

Obesity (2016) and its 6 proposals to address the obesogenic condition and basic periods in the existence course to handle youth heftiness. The execution intend to direct nations in making a move to actualize the proposals of the Commission was invited by the World Health Assembly in 2017.

# Indications

Stoutness is analyzed when your weight record (BMI) is 30 or higher. To decide your weight record, separate your weight in pounds by your tallness in inches squared and duplicate by 703. Or then again partition your weight in kilograms by your tallness in meters squared.

| **BMI** | **Weight status** |
|---|---|
| Below 18.5 | Underweight |
| 18.5-24.9 | Normal |
| 25.0-29.9 | Obesity |
| 30.0 and higher | Obesity |

For the vast majority, BMI gives a sensible gauge of muscle versus fat. Notwithstanding, BMI doesn't legitimately gauge muscle to fat ratio, so a few people, for example, solid competitors, may have a BMI in the Weight class despite the fact that they don't have abundance muscle to fat ratio.

In case you're worried about weight-related medical issues, get some information about stoutness the executives. You and your primary care physician can assess your wellbeing hazards and examine your weight reduction alternatives.

## CAUSES

In spite of the fact that there are hereditary, conduct, metabolic and hormonal effects on body weight, stoutness happens when you take in a greater number of calories than you consume exercise and typical day by day exercises. Your body stores these overabundance calories as fat.

Most Americans' eating regimens are excessively high in calories — regularly from cheap food and unhealthy drinks. Individuals with weight may eat more calories before feeling full, feel hungry sooner, or eat more because of stress or nervousness.

## Danger factors

Stoutness ordinarily results from a blend of causes and contributing components:

## Family legacy and impacts

The qualities you acquire from your folks may influence the measure of muscle versus fat you store, and where that fat is disseminated. Hereditary qualities may likewise assume a part in how productively your body changes over food into vitality, how your body manages your craving and how your body consumes calories during exercise.

Weight will in general altercation families. That is not a direct result of the qualities they share.

Relatives likewise will in general have comparable eating and movement propensities.

## Way of life decisions

- Unhealthy diet. An eating regimen that is high in calories, ailing in products of the soil, brimming with cheap food, and loaded down with unhealthy refreshments and larger than usual parts adds to weight gain.
- Liquid calories. Individuals can drink numerous calories without feeling full, particularly calories from liquor. Other fatty refreshments, for example, sugared soda pops, can add to critical weight gain.
- Inactivity. On the off chance that you have an inactive way of life, you can

without much of a stretch take in a bigger number of calories consistently than you consume exercise and routine day by day exercises. Taking a gander at PC, tablet and telephone screens is an inactive movement. The quantity of hours you spend before a screen is profoundly connected with weight gain.

## Certain ailments and drugs

In certain individuals, heftiness can be followed to a clinical reason, for example, Prader-Willi disorder, Cushing condition and different conditions. Clinical issues, for example, joint pain, additionally can prompt diminished action, which may bring about weight gain.

A few prescriptions can prompt weight gain on the off chance that you don't repay through eating regimen or action. These prescriptions incorporate a few antidepressants, hostile to seizure meds, diabetes drugs, antipsychotic meds, steroids and beta blockers.

## Social and financial issues

Social and monetary variables are connected to heftiness. Keeping away from weight is troublesome on the off chance that you don't have safe zones to walk or exercise. So also, you might not have been shown sound methods of cooking, or you might not approach more beneficial nourishments. Moreover, the individuals you invest energy with may impact your weight — you're bound to create heftiness in the event that you have companions or family members with stoutness.

## Age

Weight can happen at any age, even in small kids. Yet, as you age, hormonal changes and a less dynamic way of life increment your danger of weight. Moreover, the measure of muscle in your body will in general diminish with age. For the most part, lower bulk prompts a diminishing in digestion. These progressions additionally lessen calorie needs, and can make it harder to keep off abundance weight. On the off chance that you don't intentionally control what you eat and turn out to be all the more truly dynamic as you age, you'll probably put on weight.

## Different variables

- Pregnancy. Weight gain is regular during pregnancy. A few ladies discover this weight hard to lose after the child is conceived. This weight addition may add to the advancement of Weight in ladies. Bosom taking care of might be the most ideal choice to lose the weight picked up during pregnancy.

- Quitting smoking. Stopping smoking is frequently connected with weight gain. Furthermore, for a few, it can prompt enough weight increase to qualify as Weight. Regularly, this occurs as individuals use food to adapt to smoking withdrawal. Over the long haul, nonetheless, stopping smoking is as yet a more prominent advantage to your wellbeing than is proceeding to smoke. Your primary care physician can assist you with forestalling weight increase subsequent to stopping smoking.

- Lack of rest. Not getting enough rest or getting an excessive amount of rest can cause changes in hormones that expansion your craving. You may likewise hunger for nourishments high in calories and sugars, which can add to weight gain.

- Stress. Numerous outside elements that influence your disposition and prosperity may add to stoutness. Individuals frequently look for all the unhealthier food while encountering unpleasant circumstances.

- Microbiome. Your gut microbes are influenced by what you eat and may add to weight put on or trouble getting in shape.

- Previous endeavors to get in shape. Past endeavors of weight reduction followed by quick weight recover may add to additionally weight gain. This wonder, once in a while called yo-yo abstaining from excessive food intake, can slow your digestion.

Regardless of whether you have at least one of these danger factors, it doesn't imply that you're bound to create weight. You can check most hazard factors through eating regimen, physical movement and exercise, and conduct changes.

## Entanglements

Individuals with stoutness are bound to build up various possibly genuine medical issues, including:

- Heart sickness and strokes. Stoutness makes you bound to have hypertension and anomalous cholesterol levels, which are hazard factors for coronary illness and strokes.

- Type 2 diabetes. Weight can influence the manner in which your body utilizes insulin to control glucose levels. This raises your danger of insulin opposition and diabetes.

- Certain tumors. Weight may build your danger of malignancy of the uterus, cervix, endometrium, ovary, bosom, colon, rectum, throat, liver, gallbladder, pancreas, kidney and prostate.

- Digestive issues. Heftiness improves the probability that you'll create indigestion, gallbladder illness and liver issues.

- Gynecological and sexual issues. Heftiness may cause fruitlessness and unpredictable periods in ladies. Weight additionally can cause erectile brokenness in men.

- Sleep apnea. Individuals with Weight are bound to have rest apnea, a conceivably genuine turmoil wherein breathing over and again stops and starts during rest.

- Osteoarthritis. Stoutness expands the pressure put on weight-bearing joints, notwithstanding advancing aggravation inside the body. These elements may prompt difficulties, for example, osteoarthritis.

## Personal satisfaction

Heftiness can lessen your general personal satisfaction. You will be unable to do things you used to do, for example, partaking in charming exercises. You may evade public spots. Individuals with Weight may even experience segregation.

Other weight-related issues that may influence your personal satisfaction include:

- Depression
- Disability
- Sexual issues
- Shame and blame

- Social confinement

- Lower work accomplishment

## How to Avoid Weight and Obesity

Regardless of whether you're in danger of Weight, at present Obesity or at a solid weight, you can find a way to forestall unfortunate weight gain and related medical issues. Of course, the means to forestall weight gain are equivalent to the means to get thinner: every day work out, a sound eating routine, and a drawn-out pledge to watch what you eat and drink.

- Exercise normally. You have to get 150 to 300 minutes of moderate-force action seven days to forestall weight gain. Modestly serious physical exercises incorporate quick strolling and swimming.

- Follow a smart dieting plan. Zero in on low-calorie, supplement thick nourishments, for example, natural products, vegetables and entire grains. Dodge soaked fat and breaking point desserts and liquor. Eat three standard dinners daily with restricted nibbling. You can even now appreciate limited quantities of high-fat, fatty nourishments as a rare treat. Simply make certain to pick nourishments that advance a sound weight and great wellbeing more often than not.

- Know and dodge the food traps that cause you to eat. Recognize circumstances that trigger wild eating. Have a go at keeping a diary and record what you eat, the amount you eat, when you eat, how you're feeling and how hungry you are. Inevitably, you should see designs rise. You can prepare and create systems for taking care of these kinds of circumstances and remain in charge of your eating practices.

- Monitor your weight consistently. Individuals who gauge themselves in any event once seven days are more fruitful in keeping off abundance pounds. Checking your weight can reveal to you whether your endeavors are working and can assist you with recognizing little weight gains before they become enormous issues.

- Be predictable. Adhering to your solid weight plan during the week, on the ends of the week, and in the midst of excursion and occasions however much as could be expected builds your odds of long-haul achievement.

## Analysis

To analyze heftiness, your PCP will commonly play out a physical test and suggest a few tests.

These tests and tests by and large include:

- Taking your wellbeing history. Your primary care physician may audit your weight history, weight reduction endeavors, physical movement and exercise propensities, eating examples and hunger control, what different conditions you've had, meds, feelings of anxiety, and different issues about your wellbeing. Your PCP may likewise audit your family's wellbeing history to check whether you might be inclined to specific conditions.

- A general physical test. This incorporates estimating your tallness; checking indispensable signs, for example, pulse, circulatory strain and temperature; tuning in to your heart and lungs; and analyzing your mid-region.

- Calculating your BMI. Your primary care physician will check your weight record (BMI). A BMI of 30 or higher is viewed as Weight. Numbers higher than 30 increment your wellbeing hazards considerably more. Your BMI ought to be checked in any event once every year since it can help decide your general wellbeing hazards and what medicines might be suitable.

- Measuring your abdomen circuit. Fat put away around your midsection, once in a while called instinctive fat or stomach fat, may additionally build your danger of coronary illness and diabetes. Ladies with an abdomen estimation (circuit) of in excess of 35 inches (89 centimeters, or cm) and men with a midriff estimation of in excess of 40 inches (102 cm) may have more wellbeing hazards than do individuals with littler midsection estimations. Like the BMI estimation, your midsection periphery ought to be checked at any rate once per year.

- Checking for other medical issues. In the event that you have known medical issues, your PCP will assess them. Your PCP will likewise check for other conceivable medical issues, for example, hypertension and diabetes. Your PCP may likewise suggest certain heart tests, for example, an electrocardiogram.

- Blood tests. What tests you have rely upon your wellbeing, hazard factors and any current indications you might be having. Blood tests may incorporate a cholesterol test, liver capacity tests, a fasting glucose, a thyroid test and others.

Assembling this data encourages you and your PCP decide how much weight you have to lose and what wellbeing conditions or dangers you as of now have. Also, this will manage treatment choices.

**How To Treat Weight and Obesity**

The objective of stoutness treatment is to reach and remain at a solid weight. This improves your general wellbeing and brings down your danger of creating difficulties identified with Weight. You may need to work with a group of wellbeing experts — including a dietitian, social advisor or a weight authority — to assist you with comprehension and make changes in your eating and action propensities.

The underlying treatment objective is typically a humble weight reduction — 5% to 10% of your absolute weight. That implies that on the off chance that you weigh 200 pounds (91 kg) and have stoutness by BMI guidelines, you would need to lose just around 10 to 20 pounds (4.5 to 9 kg) for your wellbeing to start to improve. Be that as it may, the more weight you lose, the more noteworthy the advantages.

All health improvement plans require changes in your dietary patterns and expanded physical action. The treatment techniques that are directly for you rely upon your heftiness seriousness, your general wellbeing and your readiness to take an interest in your weight reduction plan.

## Dietary changes

Lessening calories and rehearsing more beneficial dietary patterns are crucial to defeating heftiness. Despite the fact that you may get in shape rapidly from the outset, consistent weight reduction over the long haul is viewed as the most secure approach to get more fit and the most ideal approach to keep it off for all time.

Dodge exceptional and ridiculous eating routine changes, for example, crash slims down, in light of the fact that they're probably not going to assist you with keeping overabundance weight off as long as possible.

Plan to partake in a thorough health improvement plan for in any event a half year and in the upkeep period of a program for at any rate a year to support your chances of weight reduction achievement.

There is no best weight reduction diet. Pick one that incorporates solid nourishments that you feel will work for you. Dietary changes to treat stoutness include:

- **Cutting calories.** The way to weight reduction is decreasing the number of calories you take in. The initial step is to survey your run of the mill eating and drinking propensities to perceive the number of calories you regularly devour and where you can scale back. You and your primary care physician can choose the number of calories you have to take in every day to shed pounds, yet a normal sum is 1,200 to 1,500 calories for ladies and 1,500 to 1,800 for men.

- **Feeling full on less.** A few nourishments —, for example, sweets, confections, fats and handled food sources — contain a lot of calories for a little part. Conversely, foods grown from the ground furnish a bigger bit size with less calories. By eating bigger bits of nourishments that have less calories, you decrease cravings for food, take in less calories and rest easy thinking about your supper, which adds to how fulfilled you feel by and large.

- **Making more advantageous decisions.** To make your general eating routine more advantageous, eat more plant-based nourishments, for example, natural products, vegetables and entire grain starches. Additionally stress lean wellsprings of protein —, for example, beans, lentils and soy — and lean meats. On the off chance that you like fish, attempt to incorporate fish two times per week. Breaking point salt and included sugar. Eat modest quantities of fats, and ensure they originate from heart-sound sources, for example, olive, canola and nut oils.

- **Restricting certain nourishments.** Certain eating regimens limit the measure of a specific nutrition class, for example, high-starch or full-fat nourishments. Ask your PCP which diet plans have been discovered viable and which may be useful for you. Drinking sugar-improved refreshments is a certain method to devour a greater number of calories than you expected, and restricting these beverages or killing them by and large is a decent spot to begin cutting calories.

- **Meal substitutions.** These plans propose that you supplant a couple of dinners with their items —, for example, low-calorie shakes or supper bars — and eat well bites and a solid, adjusted third feast that is low in fat and calories. Temporarily, this kind of diet can assist you with shedding pounds. Remember that these eating regimens probably won't show you how to change your general way of life, however, so you may need to keep this up in the event that you need to keep your weight off.

Be careful about convenient solutions. You might be enticed by craze consumes less calories that guarantee quick and simple weight reduction. The truth, in any case, is that there are no enchantment nourishments or convenient solutions. Prevailing fashion diets may help temporarily, yet the drawn-out outcomes don't seem, by all accounts, to be any superior to different eating regimens.

So also, you may get more fit on an accident diet, yet you're probably going to recover it when you stop the eating routine. To get thinner — and keep it off — you need to receive good dieting propensities that you can keep up after some time.

**Exercise and action**

Expanded physical action or exercise is a basic piece of Weight treatment. The vast majority who can keep up their weight reduction for over a year get ordinary exercise, even basically strolling.

To help your action level:

- **Exercise.** Individuals with Weight need to get in any event 150 minutes per seven day stretch of moderate-force physical movement to forestall further weight gain or to keep up the departure of an unassuming measure of weight. To accomplish more-noteworthy weight reduction, you may need to practice 300 minutes or more seven days. You likely should bit by bit build the sum you practice as your continuance and wellness improve.

- **Keep moving.** Despite the fact that ordinary vigorous exercise is the most proficient approach to consume calories and shed overabundance weight, any additional development helps consume calories. Rolling out basic improvements during your time can indicate huge advantages. Park farther from store passages, fire up your family tasks, garden, get up and move around occasionally, and wear a pedometer to follow the number of steps you really assume control throughout a day. A pleasant prescribed objective is to attempt to arrive at 10,000 stages each day. Progressively increment the measure of steps to arrive at that objective.

**Conduct changes**

A conduct adjustment program can assist you with making way of life changes and get more fit and keep it off. Steps to take incorporate looking at your present propensities to discover what elements, stresses or circumstances may have added to your Weight.

Everybody is unique and has various hindrances to overseeing weight, for example, an absence of time to practice or late-evening eating. Tailor your conduct changes to address your individual concerns.

Conduct alteration, some of the time called conduct treatment, can include:

- **Counseling.** Chatting with a psychological well-being proficient can assist you with tending to passionate and social issues identified with eating. Treatment can assist you with understanding why you indulge and learn solid approaches to adapt to uneasiness. You can likewise figure out how to screen your eating regimen and movement, comprehend eating triggers, and adapt to food yearnings. Advising can be one-on-one or in a gathering. More-escalated programs — those that incorporate 12 to 26 meetings per year — might be more useful in accomplishing your weight reduction objectives.

- **Support gatherings.** You can discover kinship and comprehension in help bunches where others share comparable difficulties with weight. Check with your PCP, neighborhood emergency clinics or business health improvement plans for help bunches in your general vicinity.

# Remedy weight reduction prescription

Getting thinner requires a solid eating regimen and customary exercise. However, in specific circumstances, remedy weight reduction medicine may help.

Remember, however, that weight reduction medicine is intended to be utilized alongside diet, exercise and conduct changes, not rather than them. The fundamental reason for weight reduction prescriptions, otherwise called enemy of heftiness drugs, is to assist you with adhering to a low-calorie diet by halting the yearning and absence of completion flags that show up when attempting to get thinner.

Your PCP may suggest weight reduction drug if other eating routine and exercise programs haven't worked and you meet one of these rules:

- Your weight file (BMI) is 30 or more prominent
- Your BMI is more prominent than 27, and you additionally have clinical inconveniences of Weight, for example, diabetes, hypertension or rest apnea

Before choosing a prescription for you, your PCP will think about your wellbeing history, as well as could be expected symptoms. Some weight reduction drugs can't be utilized by ladies who are pregnant or by individuals who take certain prescriptions or have incessant wellbeing conditions.

Against Weight meds affirmed by the Food and Drug Administration (FDA) include:

- Orlistat (Alli, Xenical)
- Phentermine and topiramate (Qsymia)
- Bupropion and naltrexone (Contrave)
- Liraglutide (Saxenda, Victoza)

You'll require close clinical checking while at the same time assuming a remedy weight reduction prescription. Additionally, remember that a weight reduction drug may not work for everybody, and the impacts may fade after some time. At the point when you quit assuming a weight reduction prescription, you may recapture a lot or the entirety of the weight you lost.

# Endoscopic techniques for weight reduction

These sorts of methodology don't need any entry points in your skin. After you get sedation, adaptable cylinders and instruments are embedded through your mouth and down your throat into your stomach.

There are a few distinct sorts of endoscopic strategies utilized for weight reduction. One methodology includes putting join in your stomach to decrease its size and the measure of food you can serenely expend. In another endoscopic methodology, specialists embed a little inflatable into your stomach. The inflatable is loaded up with water to diminish the measure of room accessible in your stomach. This encourages you feel fuller quicker.

These systems are normally endorsed for individuals with BMIs of 30 or above when diet and exercise alone have not been fruitful. The normal weight reduction changes among methods from 5% to 20% of complete body weight reduction.

## Weight reduction medical procedure

In certain individuals, weight reduction medical procedure, likewise called bariatric medical procedure, is an alternative. Weight reduction medical procedure restricts the measure of food you're ready to easily eat or diminishes the assimilation of food and calories, or it does both. While weight reduction medical procedure offers the most obvious opportunity with regards to losing the most weight, it can present genuine dangers.

Weight reduction medical procedure for stoutness might be thought of on the off chance that you have attempted different strategies to get in shape that haven't worked and:

- You have outrageous heftiness (BMI of 40 or higher)

- Your BMI is 35 to 39.9, and you likewise have a genuine weight-related medical issue, for example, diabetes or hypertension
- You're focused on making the way of life changes that are important for medical procedure to work

Weight reduction medical procedure causes a few people lose as much as 35% or a greater amount of their overabundance body weight. In any case, weight reduction medical procedure isn't a wonder heftiness fix.

It doesn't ensure that you'll lose the entirety of your abundance weight or that you'll keep it off long haul. Weight reduction accomplishment after medical procedure relies upon your pledge to rolling out long lasting improvements in your eating and exercise propensities.

Basic weight reduction medical procedures include:

- Gastric sidestep medical procedure. In gastric detour (Roux-en-Y gastric detour), the specialist makes a little pocket at the head of your stomach. The small digestive system is then stopped a separation beneath the fundamental stomach and associated with the new pocket. Food and fluid stream straightforwardly from the pocket into this aspect of the digestive system, bypassing the vast majority of your stomach.
- Adjustable gastric banding. In this strategy, your stomach is isolated into two pockets with an inflatable band. Pulling the band tight, similar to a belt, the specialist makes a small channel between the two pockets. The band shields the opening from extending and

is commonly intended to remain set up for all time.

- Biliopancreatic preoccupation with duodenal switch. This technique starts with the specialist eliminating an enormous aspect of the stomach. The specialist leaves the valve that discharges food to the small digestive system and the initial segment of the small digestive tract (duodenum). At that point the specialist deters the center segment of the digestive system and joins the last part straightforwardly to the duodenum. The isolated segment of the digestive tract is reattached to the furthest limit of the digestive system to permit bile and stomach related juices to stream into this aspect of the digestive system.
- Gastric sleeve. In this strategy, some portion of the stomach is taken out,

making a littler repository for food. It's a less convoluted medical procedure than gastric detour or biliopancreatic redirection with duodenal switch.

## Different medicines for weight and Obesity

Vagal nerve bar is another treatment for weight. It includes embedding a gadget under the skin of the midsection that sends discontinuous electrical heartbeats to the stomach vagus nerve, which tells the mind when the stomach feels vacant or full. This new innovation got FDA endorsement in 2014 for use by grown-ups who have not had the option to get in shape with a get-healthy plan and who have a BMI of 35 to 45 with in any event one stoutness related condition, for example, type 2 diabetes.

## Forestalling weight recapture after heftiness treatment

Tragically, it's not unexpected to recover weight regardless of what heftiness treatment techniques you attempt. In the event that you assume weight reduction prescriptions, you'll most likely recover weight when you quit taking them. You may even recover weight after weight reduction medical procedure on the off chance that you keep on gorging or revel in fatty nourishments or unhealthy drinks.

Perhaps the most ideal approaches to forestall recovering the weight you've lost is to get ordinary physical movement. Focus on 45 to an hour daily.

Monitor your physical action in the event that it causes you remain roused and on course. As you get more fit and increase better wellbeing, converse with your PCP about what extra exercises you may have the option to do and, if fitting, how to give your action and exercise a lift.

You may consistently need to stay careful about your weight. Consolidating a more beneficial eating routine and greater action in a viable and feasible way is the most ideal approach to keep the weight you lost off as long as possible.

Assume your weight reduction and weight upkeep each day in turn and encircle yourself with strong assets to help guarantee your prosperity. Locate a more advantageous method of living that you can stay with as long as possible.

## Clinical preliminaries

Investigate Mayo Clinic examines testing new medicines, mediations and tests as a way to forestall, distinguish, treat or deal with this infection.

## Way of life and home cures

Your push to conquer weight is bound to be fruitful on the off chance that you follow systems at home notwithstanding your conventional treatment plan. These can include:

- Learning about your condition. Instruction about stoutness can assist you with studying why you created Weight and what can be done. You may feel more engaged to take control and adhere to your treatment plan. Peruse legitimate self-improvement guides and think about talking regarding them with your primary care physician or advisor.

- **Setting sensible objectives.** At the point when you need to lose a lot of weight, you may set objectives that are unreasonable, for example, attempting to lose an excess of excessively quick. Try not to set yourself up for disappointment. Set every day or week after week objectives for exercise and weight reduction. Roll out little improvements in your eating routine as opposed to endeavoring exceptional changes that you're not prone to stay with for the long stretch.

- **Sticking to your treatment plan.** Changing a way of life, you may have lived with for a long time can be troublesome. Be straightforward with your PCP, advisor or other medical care experts in the event that you discover your movement or eating objectives slipping. You can cooperate to concoct groundbreaking thoughts or new methodologies.

- **Enlisting support.** Get your loved ones energetic about your weight reduction objectives. Encircle yourself with individuals who will uphold you and help you, not damage your endeavors. Ensure they see how significant weight reduction is to your wellbeing. You may likewise need to join a weight reduction uphold gathering.

- **Keeping a record.** Keep a food and movement log. This record can assist you with staying responsible for your eating and exercise propensities. You can find conduct that might be keeping you down and, alternately, what functions admirably for you. You can likewise utilize your log to follow other significant wellbeing boundaries, for example, pulse and cholesterol levels and in general wellness.

- **Identifying and maintaining a strategic distance from food triggers.** Divert yourself from your craving to eat with something positive, for example, calling a companion. Work on disapproving of undesirable nourishments and enormous segments. Eat when you're really eager — not just when the clock says it's an ideal opportunity to eat.

- **Taking your prescriptions as coordinated.** In the event that you assume weight reduction meds or drugs to treat stoutness related conditions, for example, hypertension or diabetes, take them precisely as recommended. On the off chance that you have an issue staying with your medicine routine or have horrendous reactions, converse with your PCP.

## Elective medication

Various dietary enhancements that guarantee to assist you with shedding weight rapidly are accessible. The adequacy, especially the drawn-out viability, and security of these items are regularly sketchy.

Natural cures, nutrients and minerals, all thought to be dietary enhancements by the

Food and Drug Administration, don't have a similar thorough testing and marking measure as over-the-counter and physician recommended meds do.

However, a portion of these substances, including items marked as "common," have drug-like impacts that can be perilous. Indeed, even a few nutrients and minerals can cause issues when taken in over the top sums. Fixings may not be standard, and they can cause capricious and unsafe reactions. Dietary enhancements can likewise cause hazardous connections with professionally prescribed meds you take. Converse with your primary care physician before taking any dietary enhancements.

Brain body treatments —, for example, needle therapy, care contemplation and yoga — may supplement other weight medicines. Be that as it may, these treatments by and large haven't been very much concentrated in the treatment of weight reduction. Converse with your PCP in case you're keen on adding a brain body treatment to your treatment.

## Adapting and backing

Converse with your PCP or advisor about improving your adapting abilities and consider these tips to adapt to stoutness and your weight reduction endeavors:

- **Journal.** Write in a diary to communicate torment, outrage, dread or different feelings.
- **Connect.** Try not to get confined. Attempt to partake in ordinary exercises and get along with family or companions intermittently.

- **Join.** Join a care group so you can associate with others confronting comparable difficulties.

- **Focus.** Remain zeroed in on your objectives. Conquering heftiness is a continuous cycle. Remain inspired by remembering your objectives. Advise yourself that you're liable for dealing with your condition and progressing in the direction of your objectives.

- **Relax.** Learn unwinding and stress the board. Figuring out how to perceive pressure and creating pressure the board and unwinding aptitudes can assist you with overseeing unfortunate dietary patterns.

**Getting ready for your arrangement**

Conversing with your PCP straightforwardly and actually about your weight concerns is perhaps the best thing you can accomplish for your wellbeing. Now and again, you might be alluded to a heftiness pro — on the off chance that one is accessible in your general vicinity. You may likewise be alluded to a social guide, dietitian or sustenance master.

## What you can do

Being a functioning member in your consideration is significant. One approach to do this is by getting ready for your arrangement. Consider your necessities and objectives for treatment. Likewise, record a rundown of inquiries to pose. These inquiries may include:

- What eating or movement propensities are likely adding to my wellbeing concerns and weight gain?

- What would i be able to do about the difficulties I face in dealing with my weight?
- Do I have other medical issues that are brought about by heftiness?
- Should I see a dietitian?
- Should I see a conduct advocate with ability in weight the board?
- What are the treatment alternatives for heftiness and my other medical issues?
- Is weight reduction mediation a possibility for me?

Make certain to tell your primary care physician about any ailments you have and about any medicine or over-the-counter prescriptions, nutrients or enhancements that you take.

## What's in store from your primary care physician

During your arrangement, your PCP is probably going to ask you various inquiries about your weight, eating, action, disposition and musings, and any side affects you may have. You might be posed such inquiries as:

- How much did you say something secondary school?
- What life occasions may have been related with weight gain?
- What and what amount do you eat in an average day?
- How much action do you get in a normal day?
- During what times of your life did you put on weight?
- What are the elements that you accept influence your weight?
- How is your day by day life influenced by your weight?
- What diets or medicines have you attempted to get in shape?

- What are your weight reduction objectives?
- Are you prepared to make changes in your way of life to shed pounds?
- What do you think may keep you from shedding pounds?

## What you can do meanwhile

On the off chance that you have time before your planned arrangement, you can help get ready for the arrangement by saving an eating routine journal for about fourteen days preceding the arrangement and by recording the number of steps you take in a day by utilizing a stage counter (pedometer).

You can likewise start to settle on decisions that will assist you with beginning to get in shape, including:

- Making solid changes in your eating routine. Incorporate more natural products, vegetables and entire grains in your eating regimen. Start to diminish divide sizes.

- Increasing your action level. Attempt to get up and move around your home all the more regularly. Start progressively in the event that you aren't fit as a fiddle or aren't accustomed to working out. Indeed, even a 10-minute every day walk can help. On the off chance that you have any wellbeing conditions or are over a particular age — more than 40 for men and more than 50 for ladies — hold up until you've conversed with your primary care physician before you start another activity program.

9 798690 550875